This book belongs

to

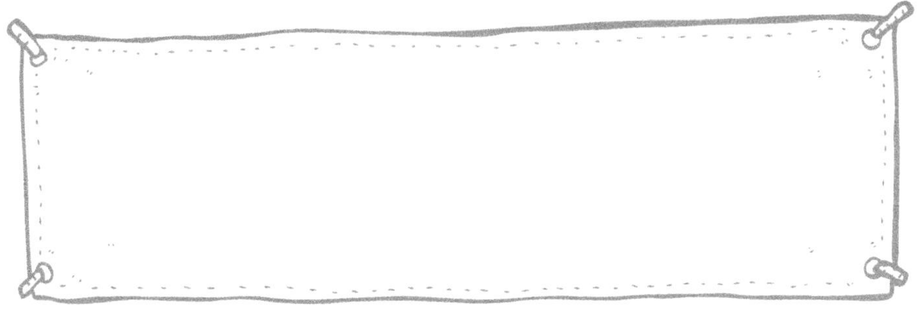

LET'S GO!

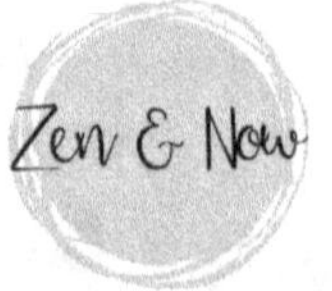
Zen & Now

How this journal works:

This journal can be used as a tool to read and to help when anxiety is high or you are in crisis.

It is a personalized collection of your happy places to help you bring feelings of calm and aid you in visualizing soothing memories. In doing so, you can greatly reduce negative feelings and emotions that can fuel your anxiety.

Drawing images can help you remember the happy moments, or you can glue pictures, swatches of material, or anything that will help you remember that event/place. There is no need to be an artist! Any image that can help you remember will do!

This journal will be a work in progress. No need to complete it all at once. You can add to it each time you experience or remember a place that brings you happiness. It can conceivably take years to conclude. However, even completing one page is a huge start in managing anxiety!

———————————— o o o ————————————

Add to this journal when you experience or remember a place that brings you joy. Refer to this journal when your anxiety is increasing. You can bring it wherever you go.

———————————— o o o ————————————

Possible examples of happy places:

- THE PARK
- THE BEACH
- FAVORITE RESTAURANT
- MY SOFA
- MY ROOM
- FLOWER FIELD
- BEING WITH MY PET
- MY BALCONY
- A PLACE IN A BOOK YOU'VE READ
- A PLACE FROM A TRIP YOU TOOK
- GOING ON A DRIVE
- GOING ON A HIKE
- FLOATING IN A POOL
- READING IN A QUIET LIBRARY
- THE POSSIBILITIES ARE ENDLESS!

Possible ideas
of your own happy places:

- ______________________________
- ______________________________
- ______________________________
- ______________________________
- ______________________________
- ______________________________
- ______________________________
- ______________________________
- ______________________________
- ______________________________
- ______________________________
- ______________________________

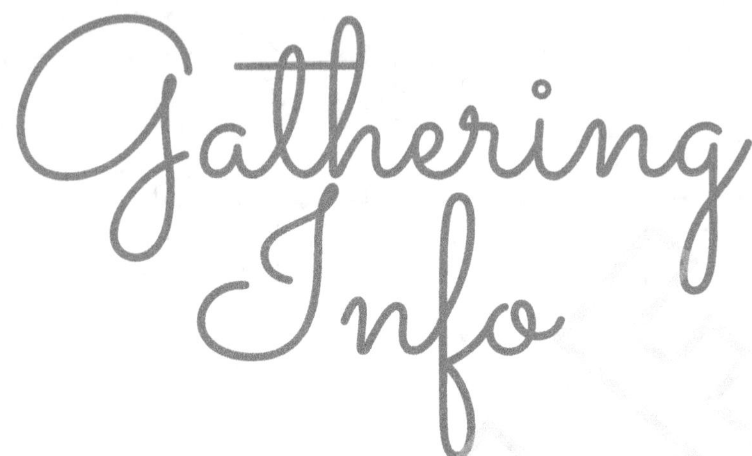

JOT DOWN WORDS ASSOCIATED WITH YOUR HAPPY PLACE
◆ YOU CAN USE SOME OR ALL OF THESE ON THE NEXT PAGE ◆

PLACE:

The Beach at Port Saint Lucie

THINGS YOU SEE

waves   sun   umbrellas   sand   pier
seagulls   frisbee   ice cream   ball

SMELLS

salty   sun cream   watermelon   fishy
cotton candy

SOUNDS

waves   people laughing   birds   wind
sand crunching under your feet   kids playing

ALL THE FEELS

wind blowing my hair   hot sun on my skin
sand on my feet and legs

The Beach at Port Saint Lucie

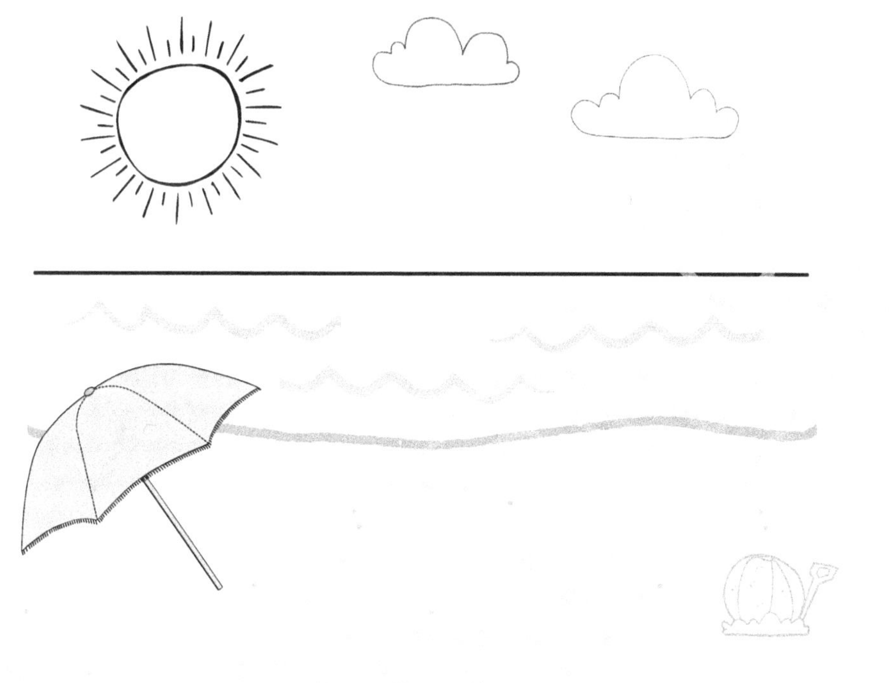

A few years ago, we went to the beach in Florida. It was such a hot and windy day. I loved how the wind felt in my hair and the sound of the waves made me feel. The water was cool, but I got used to it. I kept rinsing the sand off my feet. We brought some cold watermelon in the cooler. We walked up and down the beach and watched some kids playing with a frisbee and a hoola hoop. One man even found a horseshoe crab. We saw so many holes in the sand with bubbles coming out. Then we dug them up and found tiny crabs. I ♡ the beach!

Now it's your turn

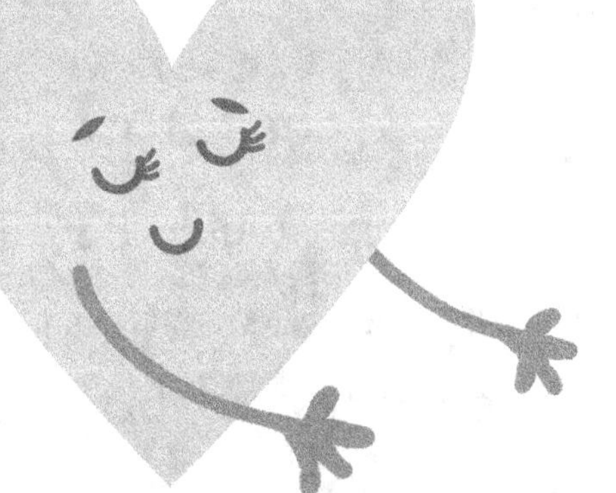

LET'S BEGIN!

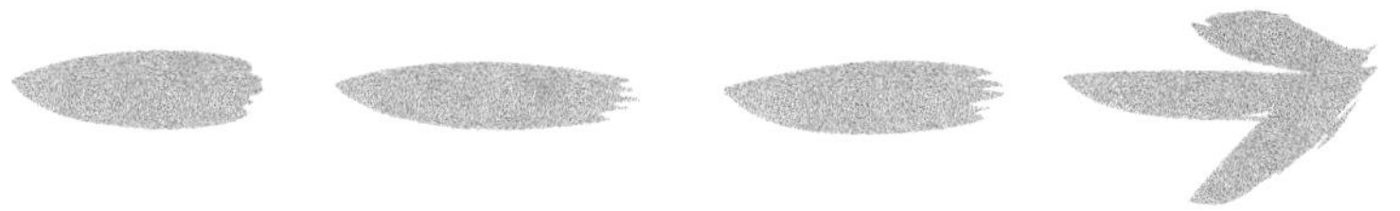

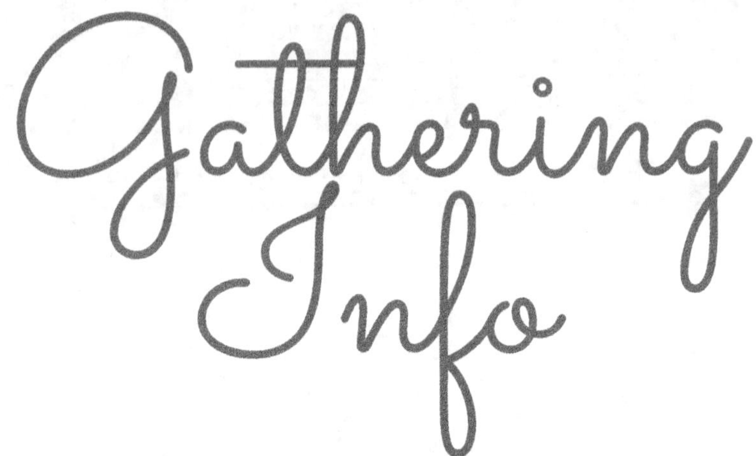

JOT DOWN WORDS ASSOCIATED WITH YOUR HAPPY PLACE
◆ YOU CAN USE SOME OR ALL OF THESE ON THE NEXT PAGE ◆

PLACE:

THINGS YOU SEE

SMELLS

SOUNDS

ALL THE FEELS

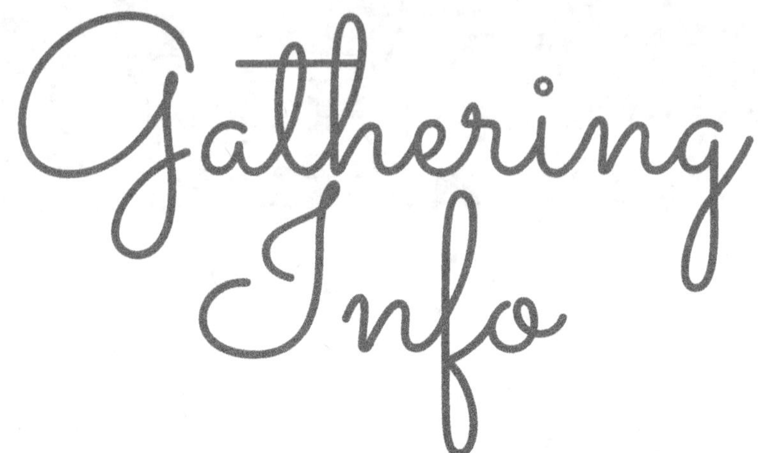

JOT DOWN WORDS ASSOCIATED WITH YOUR HAPPY PLACE
◆ YOU CAN USE SOME OR ALL OF THESE ON THE NEXT PAGE ◆

PLACE:

THINGS YOU SEE

SMELLS

SOUNDS

ALL THE FEELS

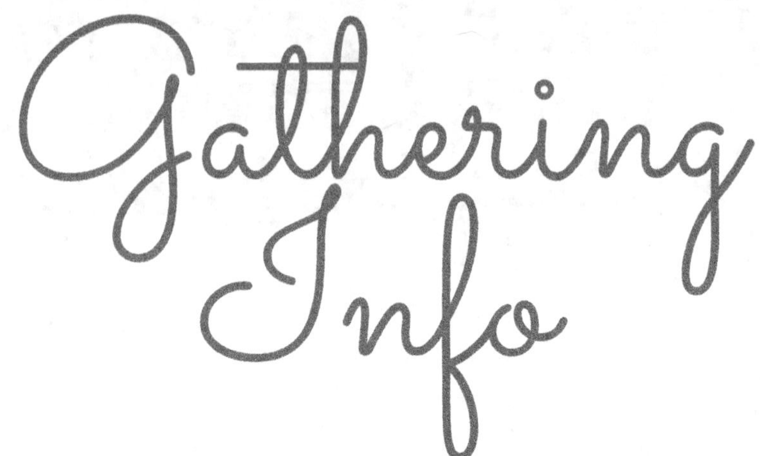

JOT DOWN WORDS ASSOCIATED WITH YOUR HAPPY PLACE
◆ YOU CAN USE SOME OR ALL OF THESE ON THE NEXT PAGE ◆

PLACE:

THINGS YOU SEE

SMELLS

SOUNDS

ALL THE FEELS

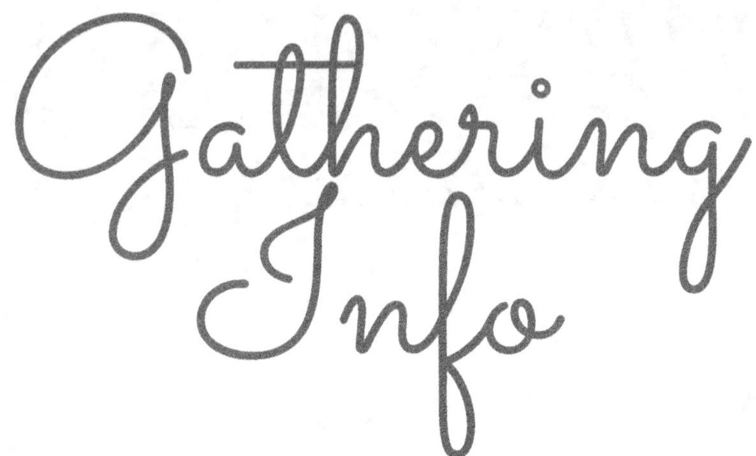

JOT DOWN WORDS ASSOCIATED WITH YOUR HAPPY PLACE
◆ YOU CAN USE SOME OR ALL OF THESE ON THE NEXT PAGE ◆

PLACE:

____

THINGS YOU SEE

____

____

SMELLS

____

____

SOUNDS

____

____

ALL THE FEELS

____

____

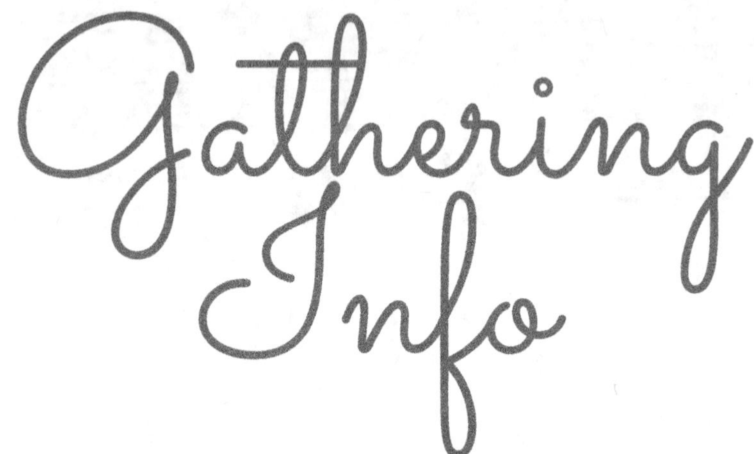

JOT DOWN WORDS ASSOCIATED WITH YOUR HAPPY PLACE
◆ YOU CAN USE SOME OR ALL OF THESE ON THE NEXT PAGE ◆

PLACE:

THINGS YOU SEE

SMELLS

SOUNDS

ALL THE FEELS

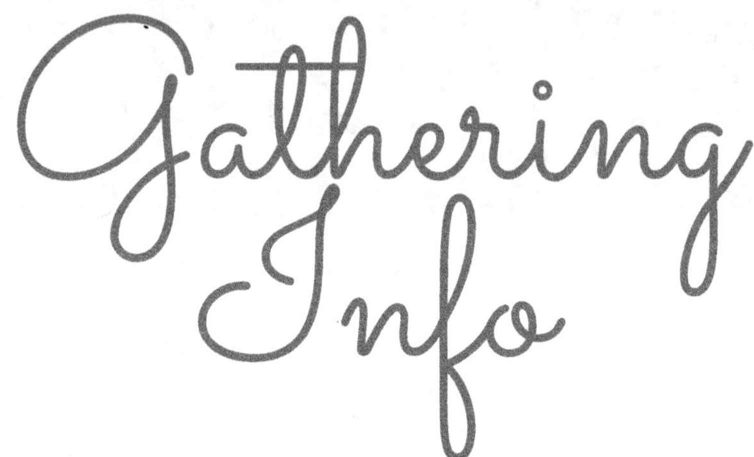

JOT DOWN WORDS ASSOCIATED WITH YOUR HAPPY PLACE

◆ YOU CAN USE SOME OR ALL OF THESE ON THE NEXT PAGE ◆

PLACE:

THINGS YOU SEE

SMELLS

SOUNDS

ALL THE FEELS

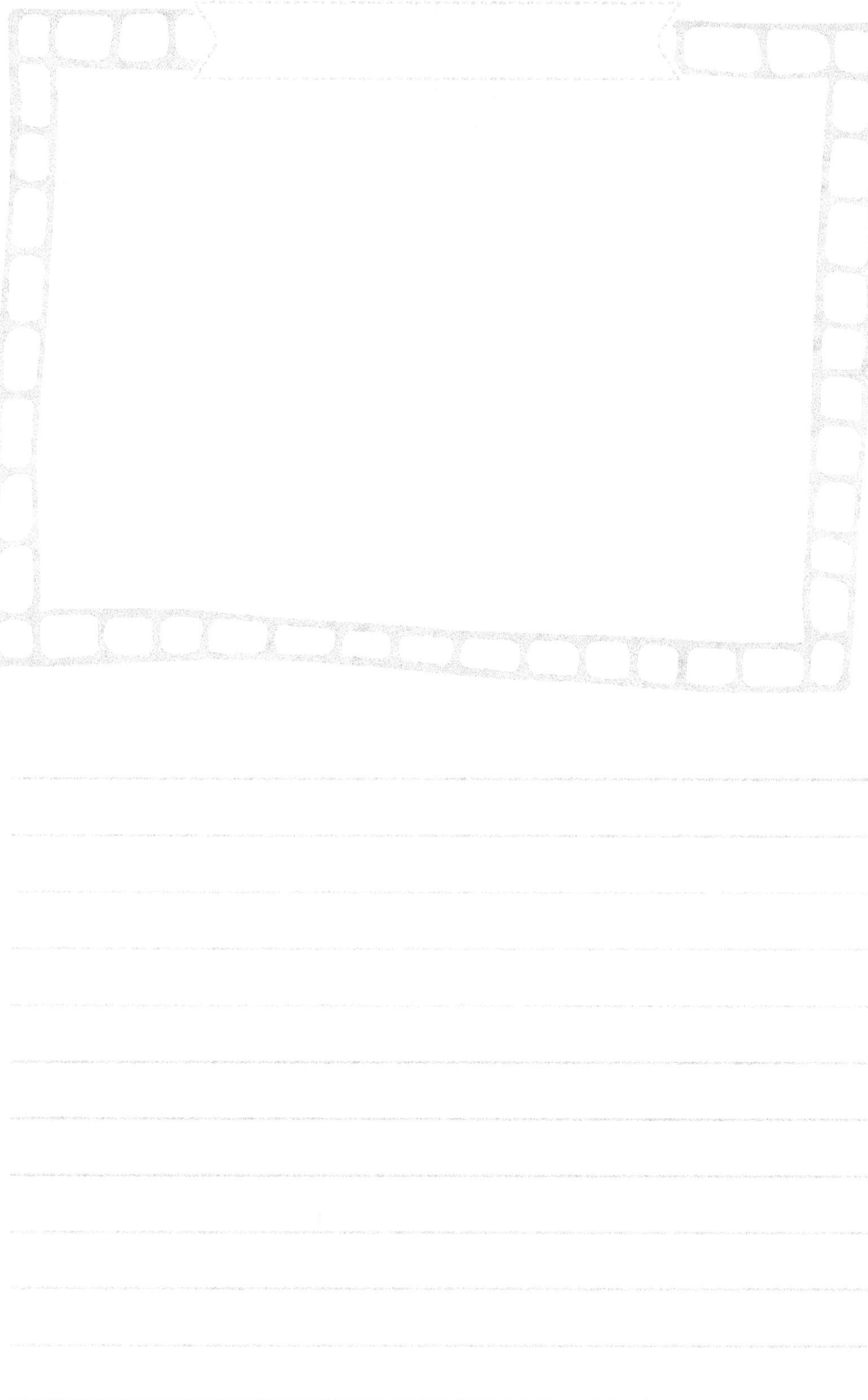

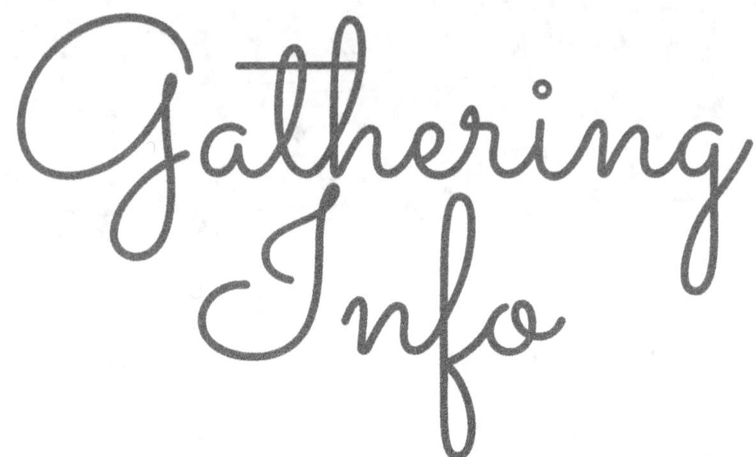

JOT DOWN WORDS ASSOCIATED WITH YOUR HAPPY PLACE
◆ YOU CAN USE SOME OR ALL OF THESE ON THE NEXT PAGE ◆

PLACE:

THINGS YOU SEE

SMELLS

SOUNDS

ALL THE FEELS

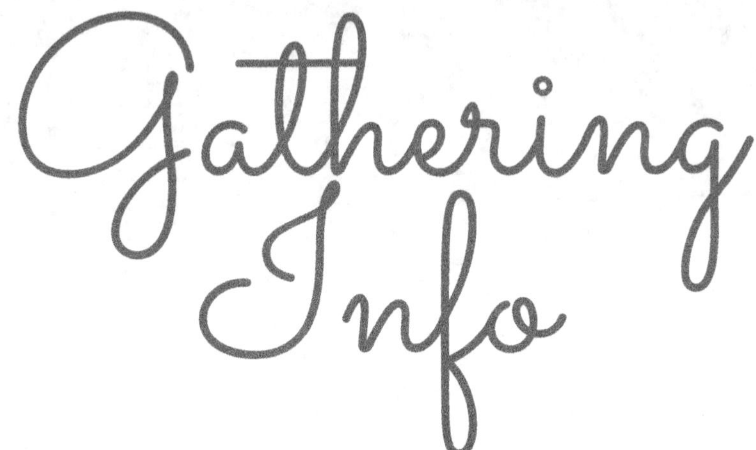

JOT DOWN WORDS ASSOCIATED WITH YOUR HAPPY PLACE
◆ YOU CAN USE SOME OR ALL OF THESE ON THE NEXT PAGE ◆

PLACE:

THINGS YOU SEE

SMELLS

SOUNDS

ALL THE FEELS

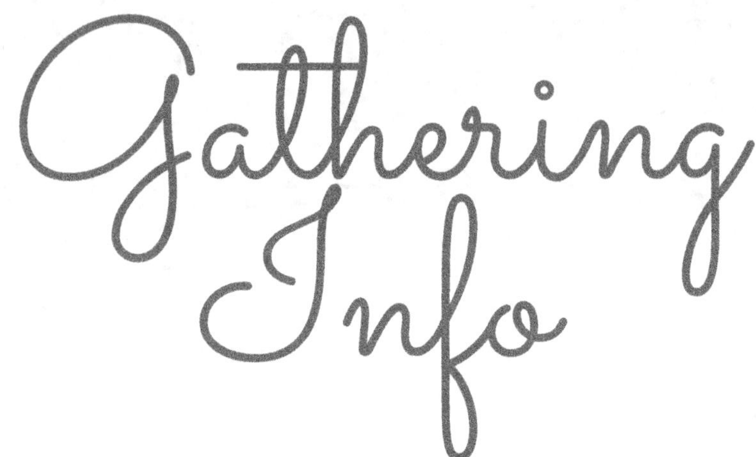

JOT DOWN WORDS ASSOCIATED WITH YOUR HAPPY PLACE
◆ YOU CAN USE SOME OR ALL OF THESE ON THE NEXT PAGE ◆

PLACE:

____

THINGS YOU SEE

____

____

SMELLS

____

____

SOUNDS

____

____

ALL THE FEELS

____

____

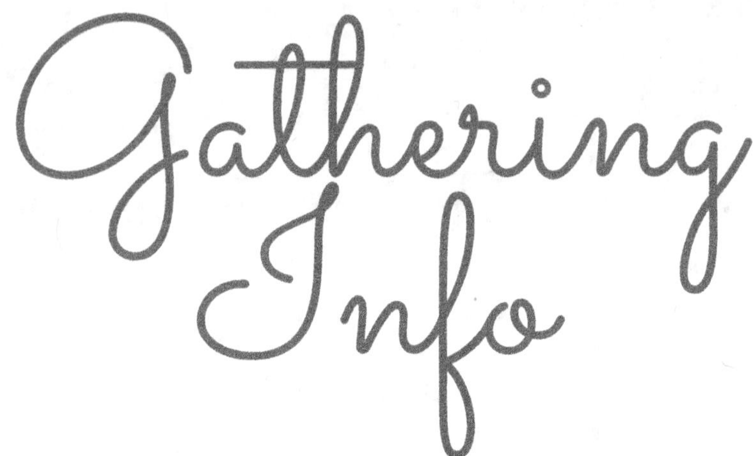

JOT DOWN WORDS ASSOCIATED WITH YOUR HAPPY PLACE
◆ YOU CAN USE SOME OR ALL OF THESE ON THE NEXT PAGE ◆

PLACE:

THINGS YOU SEE

SMELLS

SOUNDS

ALL THE FEELS

Next, some relaxing coloring

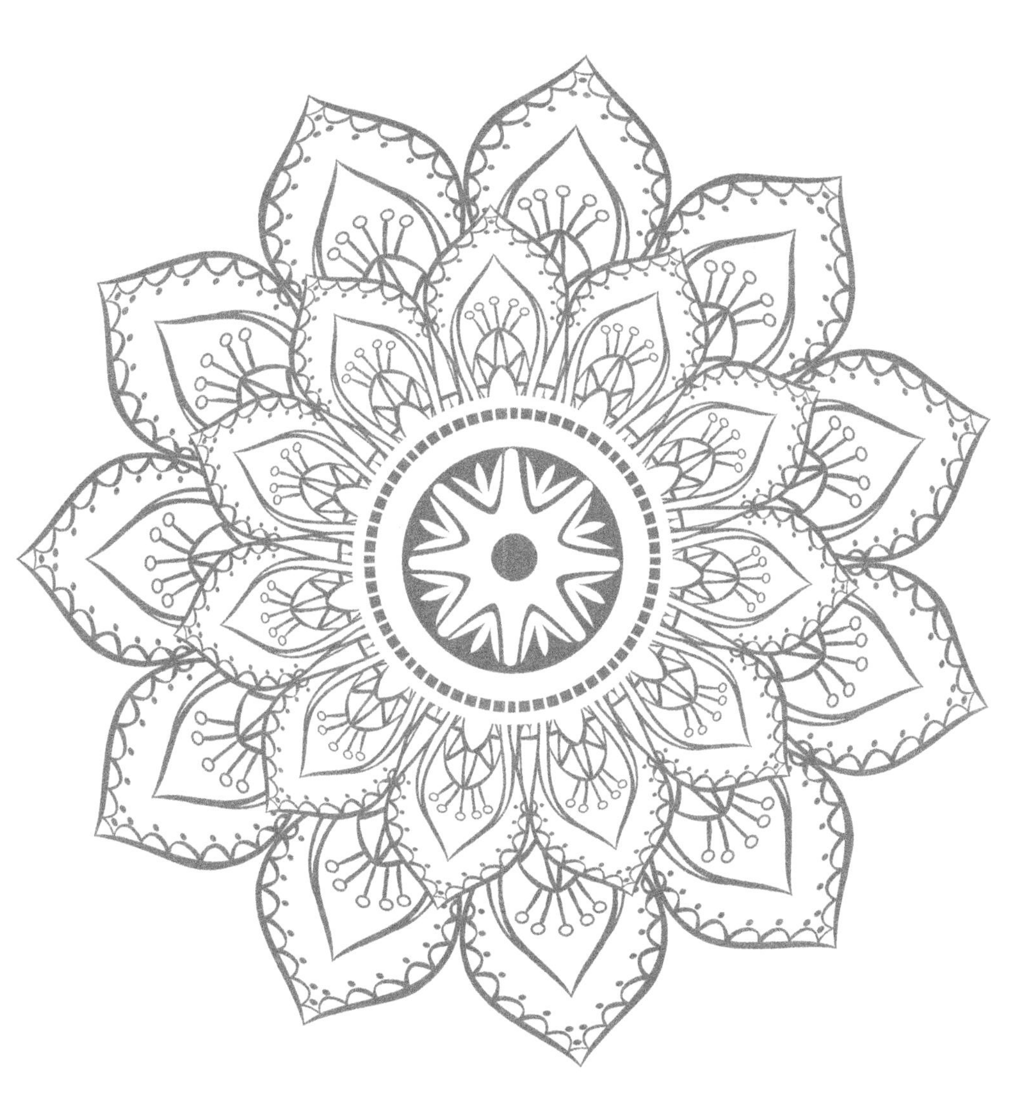

Back to more happy places

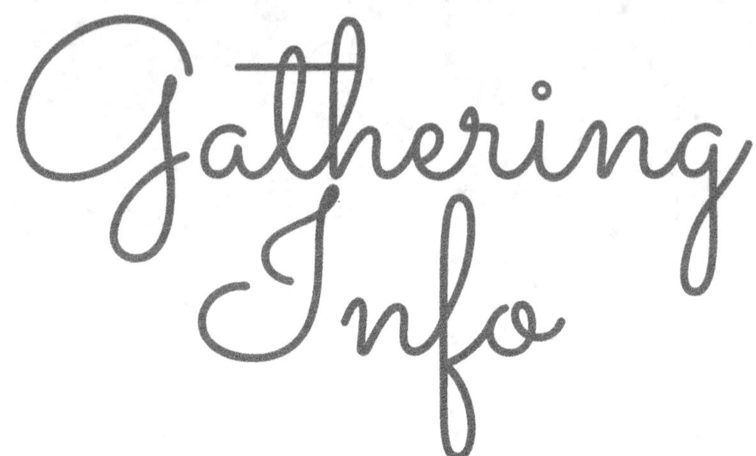

JOT DOWN WORDS ASSOCIATED WITH YOUR HAPPY PLACE
◆ YOU CAN USE SOME OR ALL OF THESE ON THE NEXT PAGE ◆

PLACE:

THINGS YOU SEE

SMELLS

SOUNDS

ALL THE FEELS

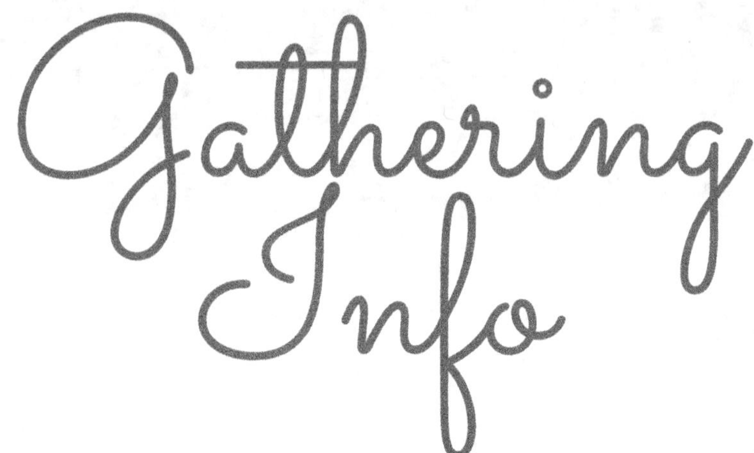

JOT DOWN WORDS ASSOCIATED WITH YOUR HAPPY PLACE
◆ YOU CAN USE SOME OR ALL OF THESE ON THE NEXT PAGE ◆

PLACE:

THINGS YOU SEE

SMELLS

SOUNDS

ALL THE FEELS

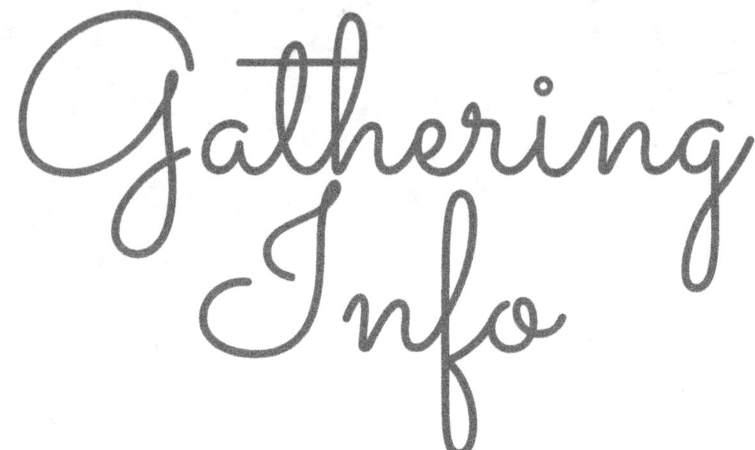

JOT DOWN WORDS ASSOCIATED WITH YOUR HAPPY PLACE
◆ YOU CAN USE SOME OR ALL OF THESE ON THE NEXT PAGE ◆

PLACE:

____

THINGS YOU SEE

____

____

SMELLS

____

____

SOUNDS

____

____

ALL THE FEELS

____

____

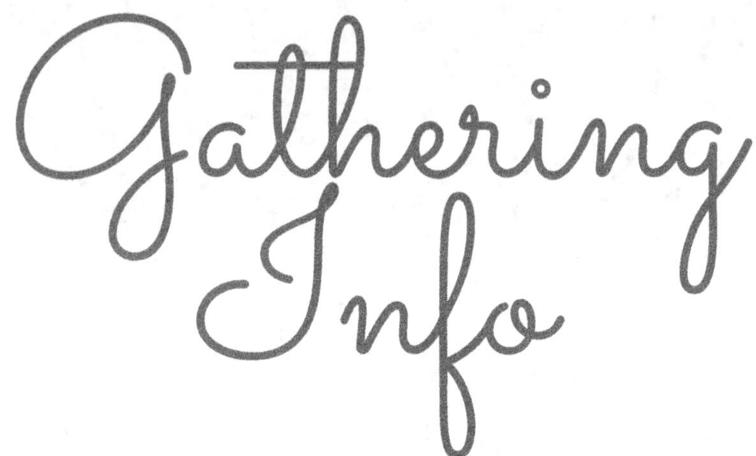

JOT DOWN WORDS ASSOCIATED WITH YOUR HAPPY PLACE
◆ YOU CAN USE SOME OR ALL OF THESE ON THE NEXT PAGE ◆

PLACE:

THINGS YOU SEE

SMELLS

SOUNDS

ALL THE FEELS

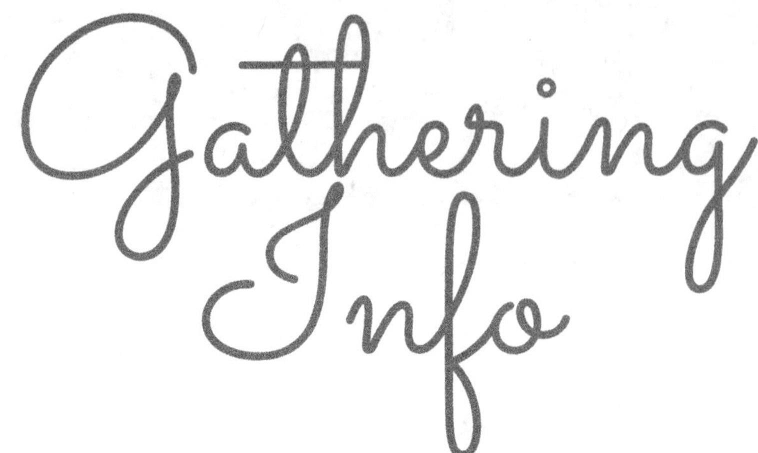

JOT DOWN WORDS ASSOCIATED WITH YOUR HAPPY PLACE

◆ YOU CAN USE SOME OR ALL OF THESE ON THE NEXT PAGE ◆

PLACE:

THINGS YOU SEE

SMELLS

SOUNDS

ALL THE FEELS

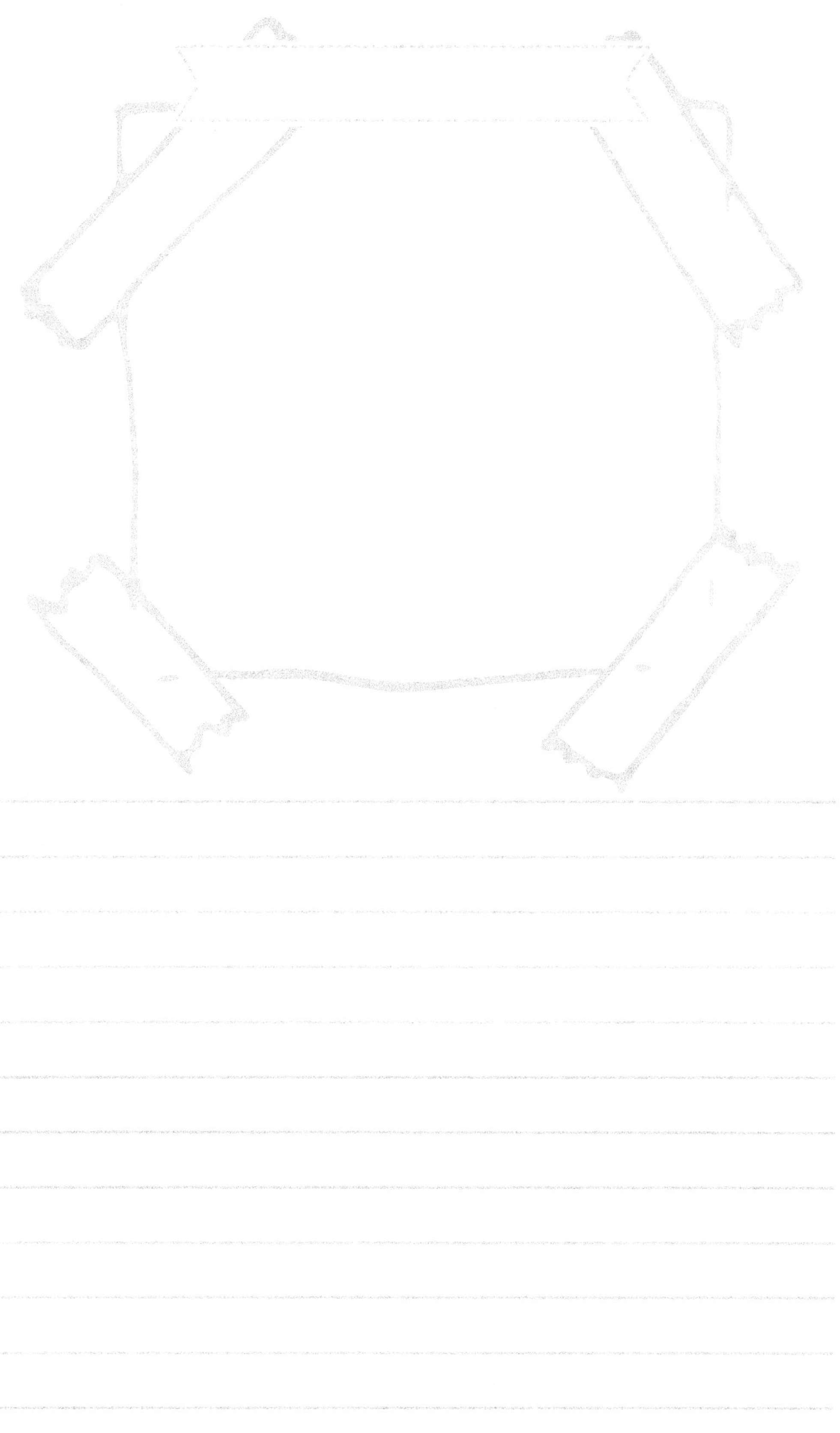

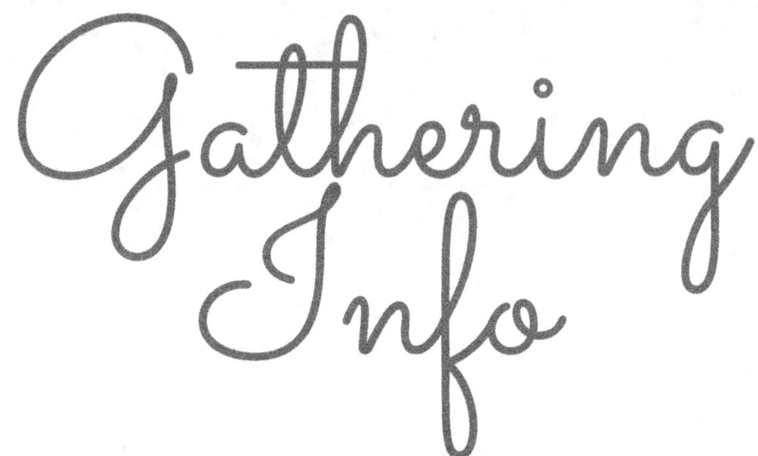

JOT DOWN WORDS ASSOCIATED WITH YOUR HAPPY PLACE
◆ YOU CAN USE SOME OR ALL OF THESE ON THE NEXT PAGE ◆

PLACE:

THINGS YOU SEE

SMELLS

SOUNDS

ALL THE FEELS

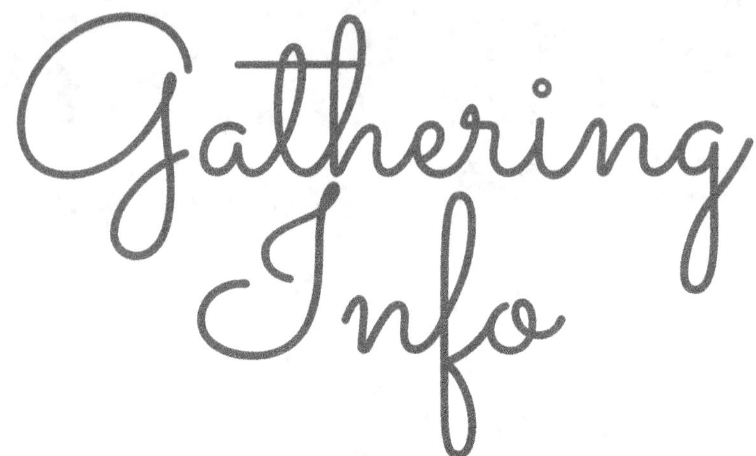

PLACE:

THINGS YOU SEE

SMELLS

SOUNDS

ALL THE FEELS

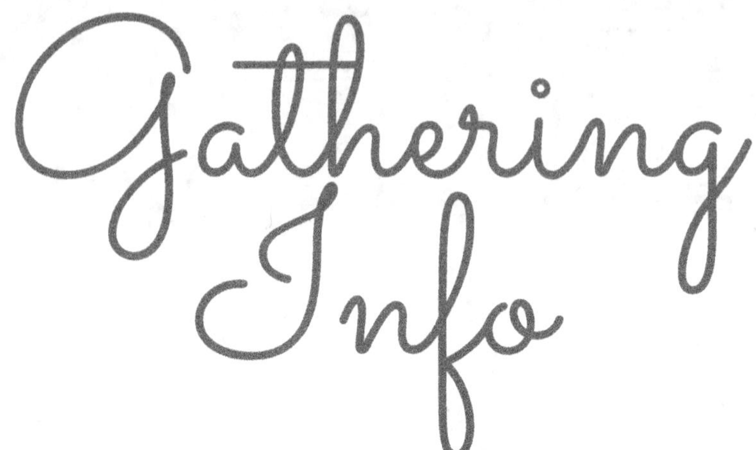

PLACE:

THINGS YOU SEE

SMELLS

SOUNDS

ALL THE FEELS

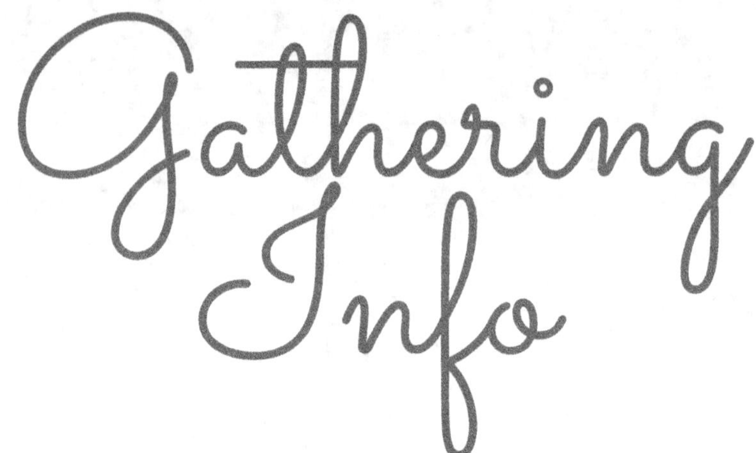

JOT DOWN WORDS ASSOCIATED WITH YOUR HAPPY PLACE
◆ YOU CAN USE SOME OR ALL OF THESE ON THE NEXT PAGE ◆

PLACE:

THINGS YOU SEE

SMELLS

SOUNDS

ALL THE FEELS

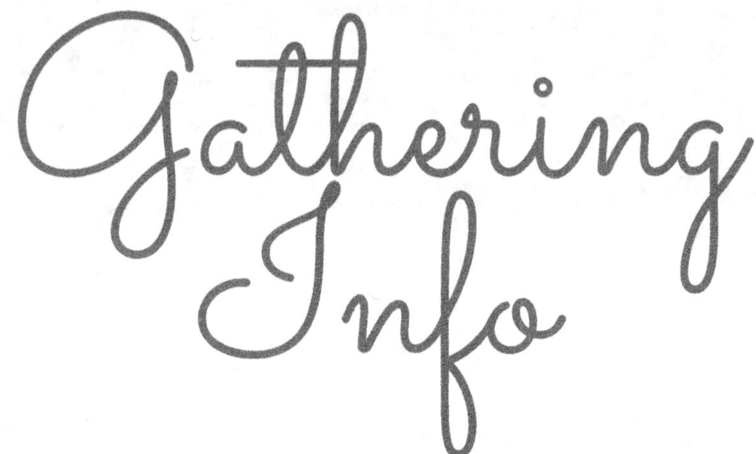

JOT DOWN WORDS ASSOCIATED WITH YOUR HAPPY PLACE
◆ YOU CAN USE SOME OR ALL OF THESE ON THE NEXT PAGE ◆

PLACE:

THINGS YOU SEE

SMELLS

SOUNDS

ALL THE FEELS

Some more relaxing coloring

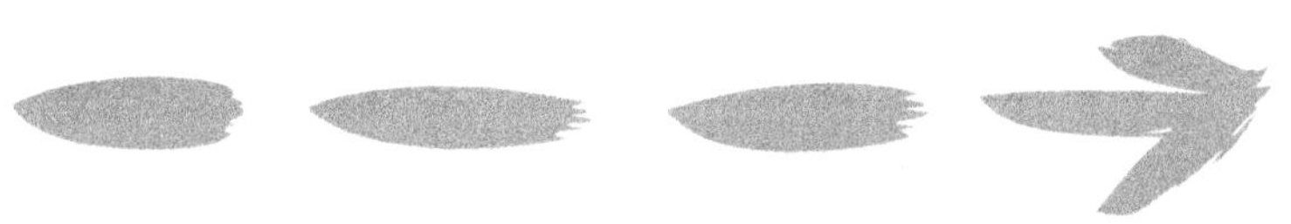

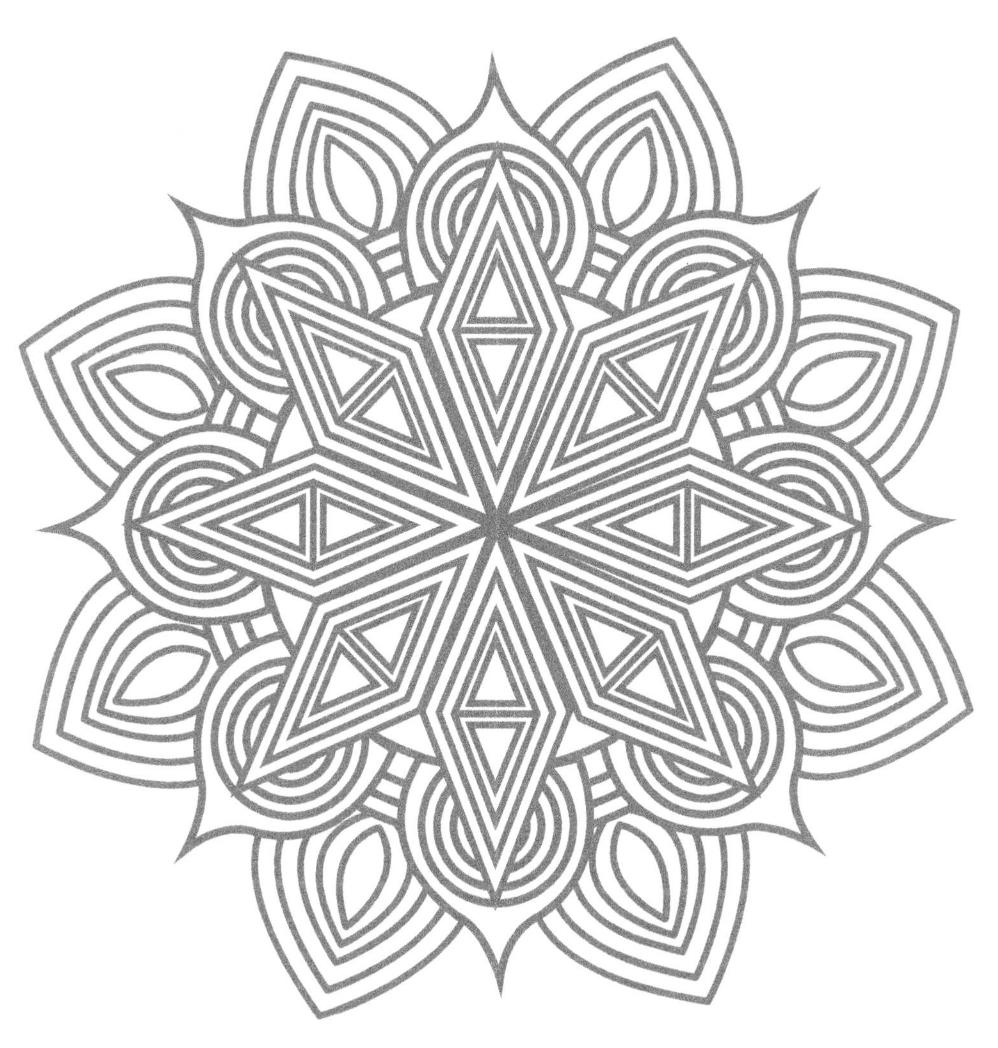

Back to more happy places

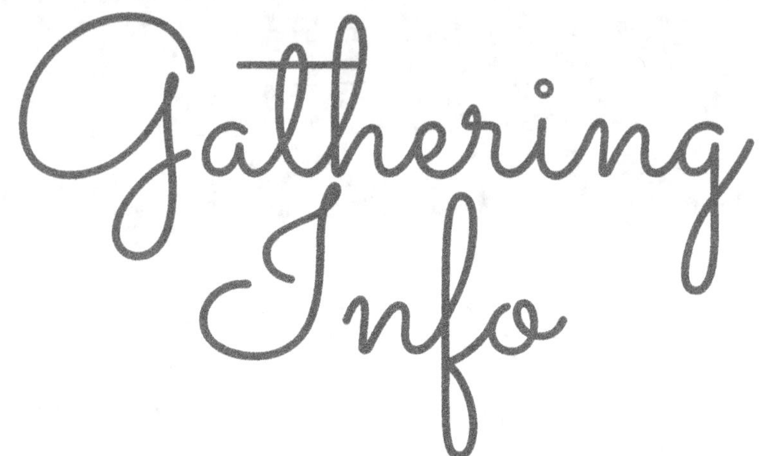

JOT DOWN WORDS ASSOCIATED WITH YOUR HAPPY PLACE
◆ YOU CAN USE SOME OR ALL OF THESE ON THE NEXT PAGE ◆

PLACE:

THINGS YOU SEE

SMELLS

SOUNDS

ALL THE FEELS

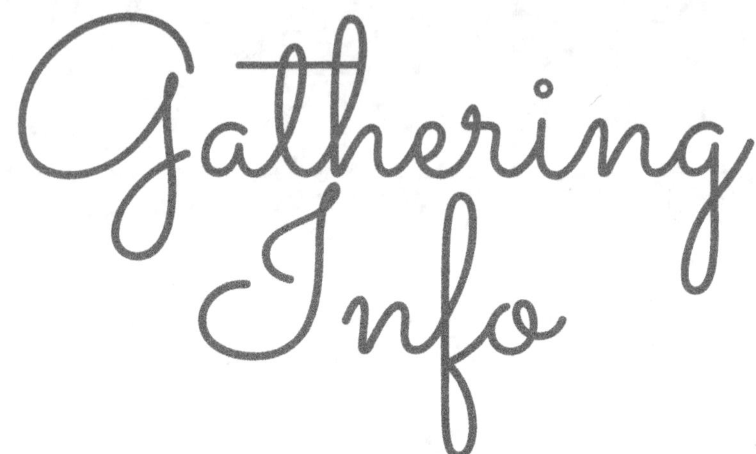

JOT DOWN WORDS ASSOCIATED WITH YOUR HAPPY PLACE
◆ YOU CAN USE SOME OR ALL OF THESE ON THE NEXT PAGE ◆

PLACE:

THINGS YOU SEE

SMELLS

SOUNDS

ALL THE FEELS

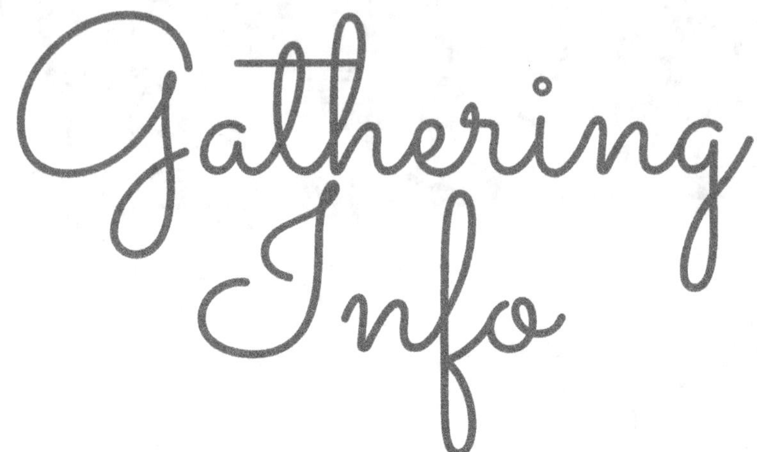

JOT DOWN WORDS ASSOCIATED WITH YOUR HAPPY PLACE
◆ YOU CAN USE SOME OR ALL OF THESE ON THE NEXT PAGE ◆

PLACE:

THINGS YOU SEE

SMELLS

SOUNDS

ALL THE FEELS

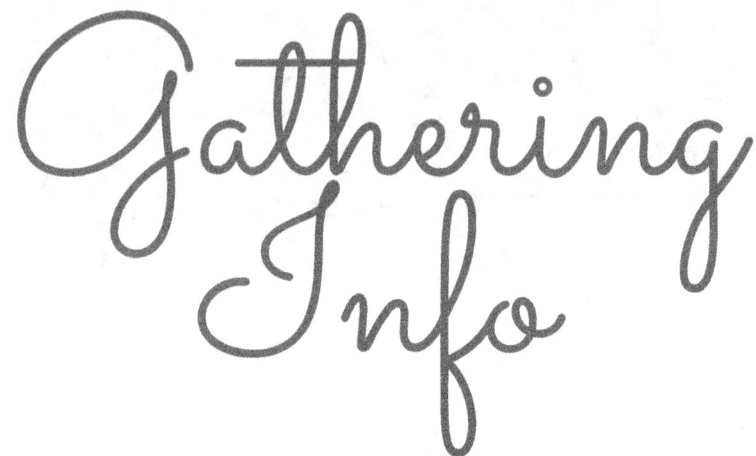

JOT DOWN WORDS ASSOCIATED WITH YOUR HAPPY PLACE
◆ YOU CAN USE SOME OR ALL OF THESE ON THE NEXT PAGE ◆

PLACE:

THINGS YOU SEE

SMELLS

SOUNDS

ALL THE FEELS

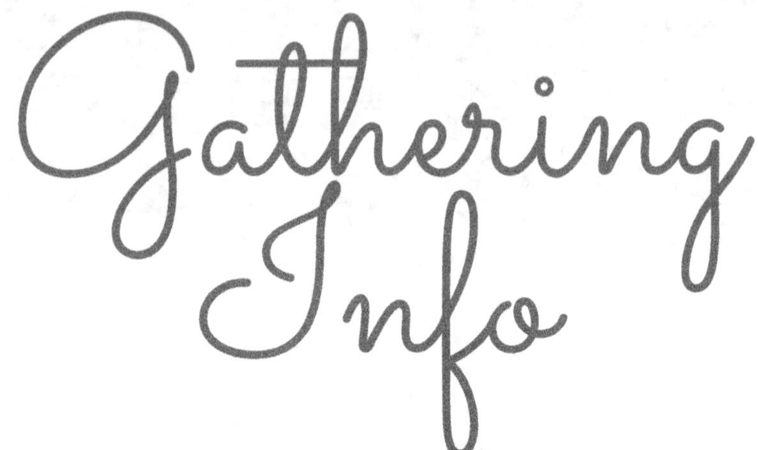

JOT DOWN WORDS ASSOCIATED WITH YOUR HAPPY PLACE
◆ YOU CAN USE SOME OR ALL OF THESE ON THE NEXT PAGE ◆

PLACE:

THINGS YOU SEE

SMELLS

SOUNDS

ALL THE FEELS

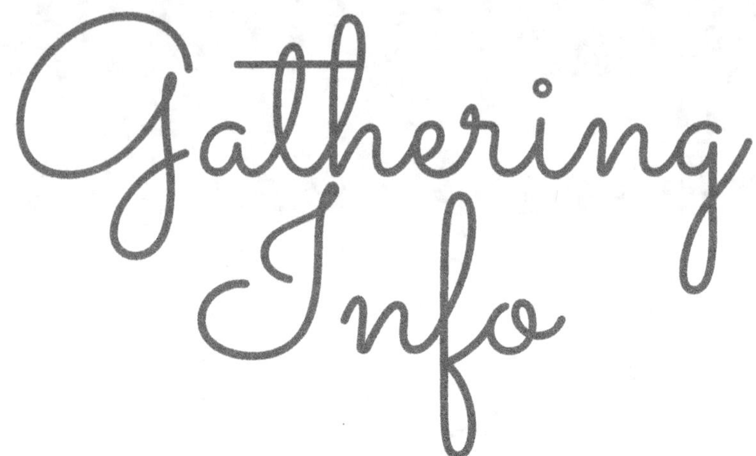

JOT DOWN WORDS ASSOCIATED WITH YOUR HAPPY PLACE
◆ YOU CAN USE SOME OR ALL OF THESE ON THE NEXT PAGE ◆

PLACE:

THINGS YOU SEE

SMELLS

SOUNDS

ALL THE FEELS

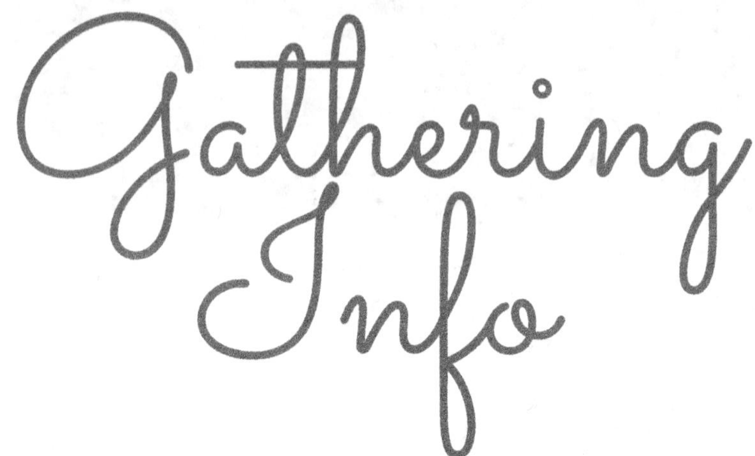

JOT DOWN WORDS ASSOCIATED WITH YOUR HAPPY PLACE
◆ YOU CAN USE SOME OR ALL OF THESE ON THE NEXT PAGE ◆

PLACE:

THINGS YOU SEE

SMELLS

SOUNDS

ALL THE FEELS

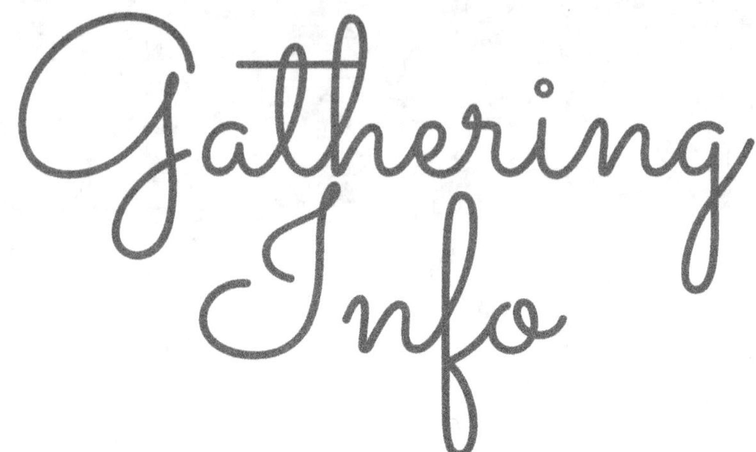

JOT DOWN WORDS ASSOCIATED WITH YOUR HAPPY PLACE
◆ YOU CAN USE SOME OR ALL OF THESE ON THE NEXT PAGE ◆

PLACE:

THINGS YOU SEE

SMELLS

SOUNDS

ALL THE FEELS

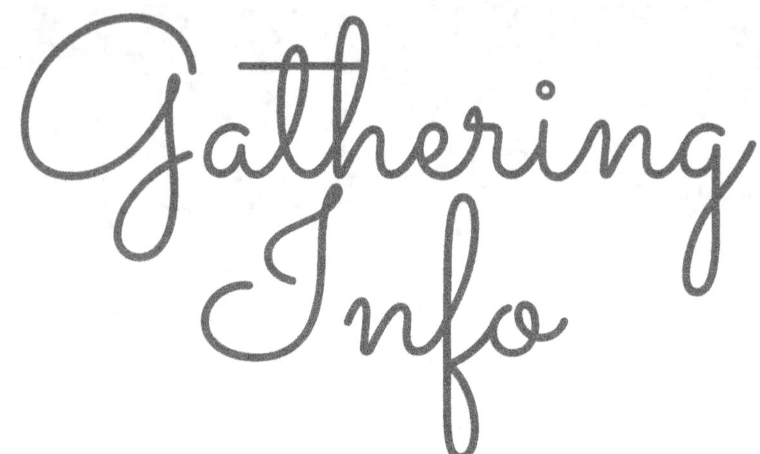

JOT DOWN WORDS ASSOCIATED WITH YOUR HAPPY PLACE
◆ YOU CAN USE SOME OR ALL OF THESE ON THE NEXT PAGE ◆

PLACE:

THINGS YOU SEE

SMELLS

SOUNDS

ALL THE FEELS

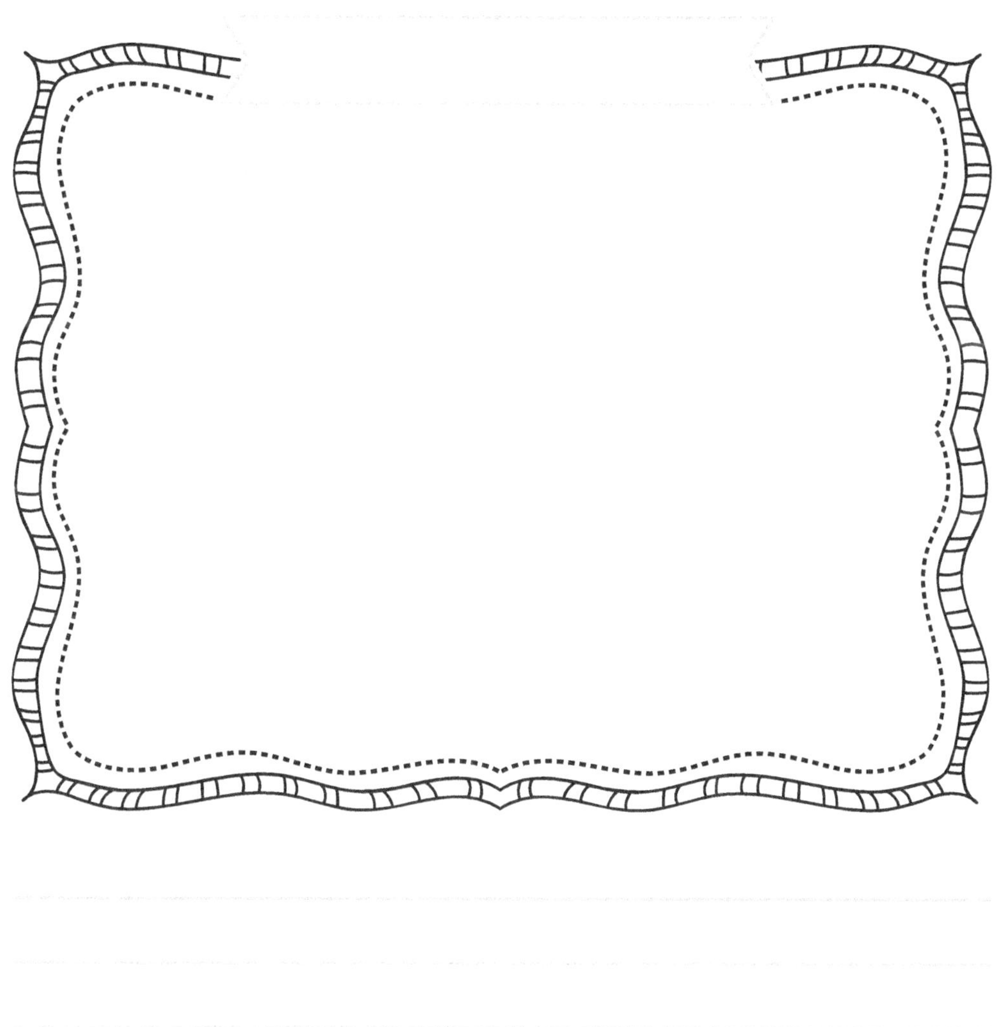

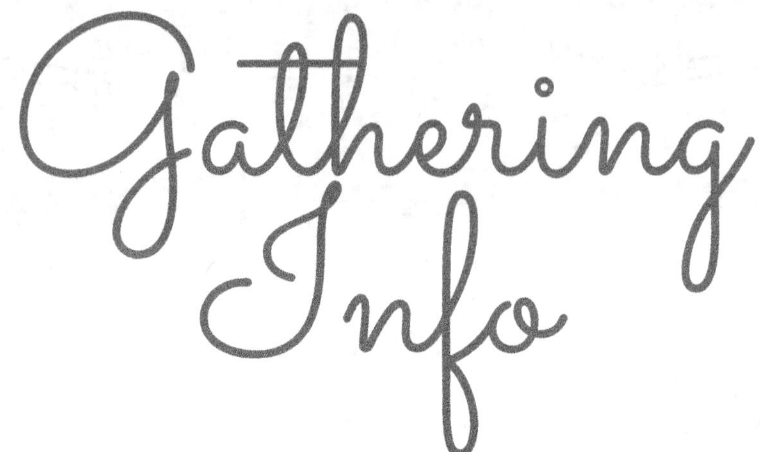

JOT DOWN WORDS ASSOCIATED WITH YOUR HAPPY PLACE
◆ YOU CAN USE SOME OR ALL OF THESE ON THE NEXT PAGE ◆

PLACE:

THINGS YOU SEE

SMELLS

SOUNDS

ALL THE FEELS

SOME MORE
RELAXING COLORING

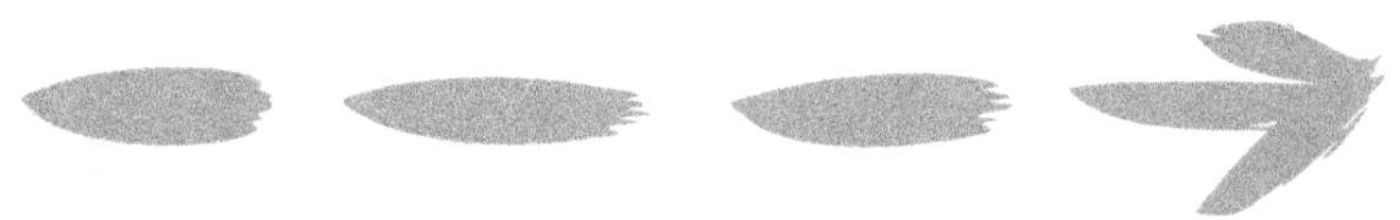

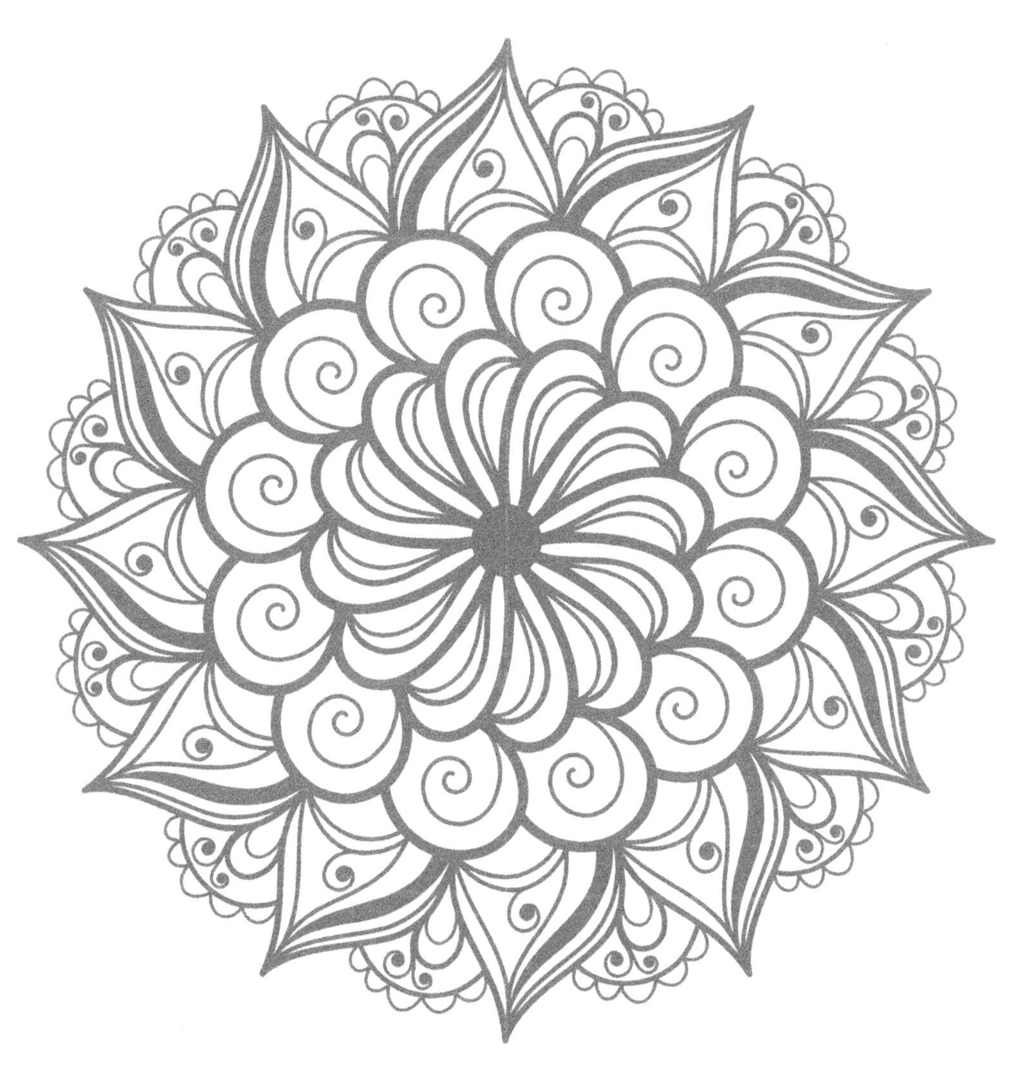

Back to more
Happy places

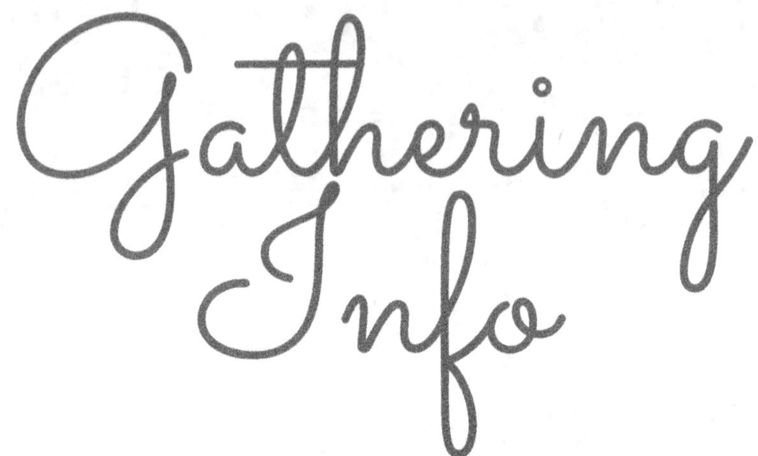

PLACE:

THINGS YOU SEE

SMELLS

SOUNDS

ALL THE FEELS

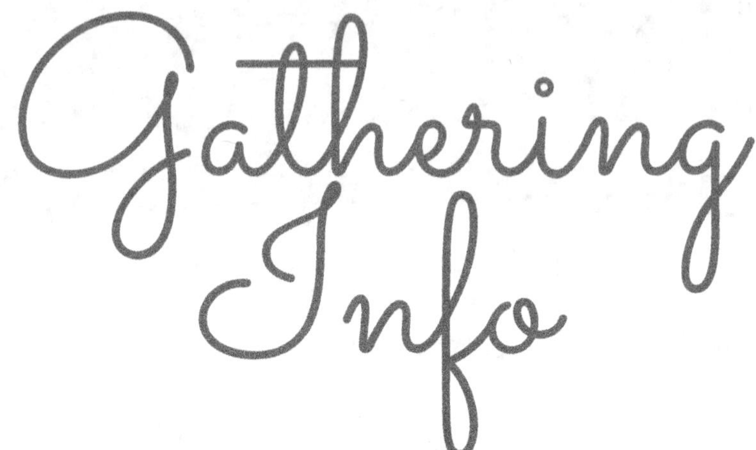

JOT DOWN WORDS ASSOCIATED WITH YOUR HAPPY PLACE
◆ YOU CAN USE SOME OR ALL OF THESE ON THE NEXT PAGE ◆

PLACE:

THINGS YOU SEE

SMELLS

SOUNDS

ALL THE FEELS

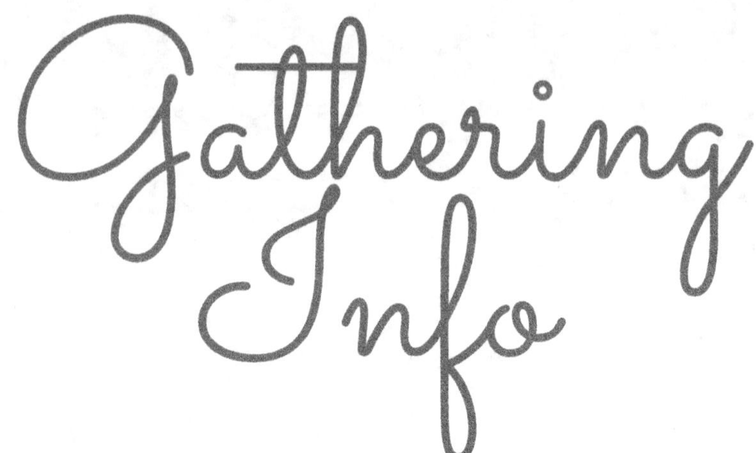

JOT DOWN WORDS ASSOCIATED WITH YOUR HAPPY PLACE
◆ YOU CAN USE SOME OR ALL OF THESE ON THE NEXT PAGE ◆

PLACE:

THINGS YOU SEE

SMELLS

SOUNDS

ALL THE FEELS

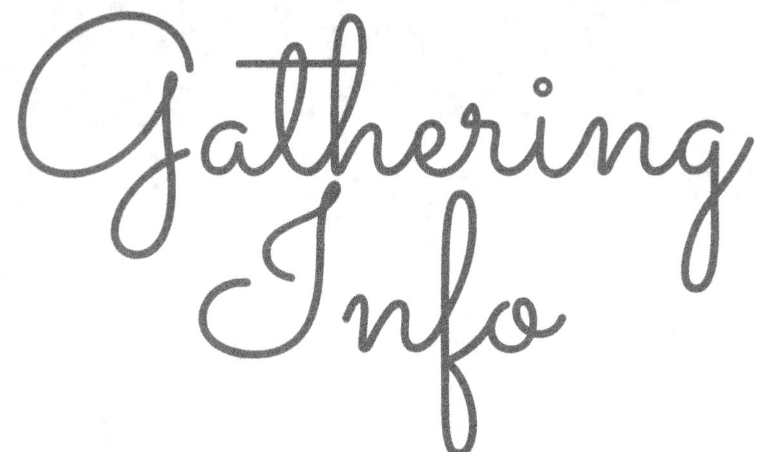

JOT DOWN WORDS ASSOCIATED WITH YOUR HAPPY PLACE
◆ YOU CAN USE SOME OR ALL OF THESE ON THE NEXT PAGE ◆

PLACE:

THINGS YOU SEE

SMELLS

SOUNDS

ALL THE FEELS

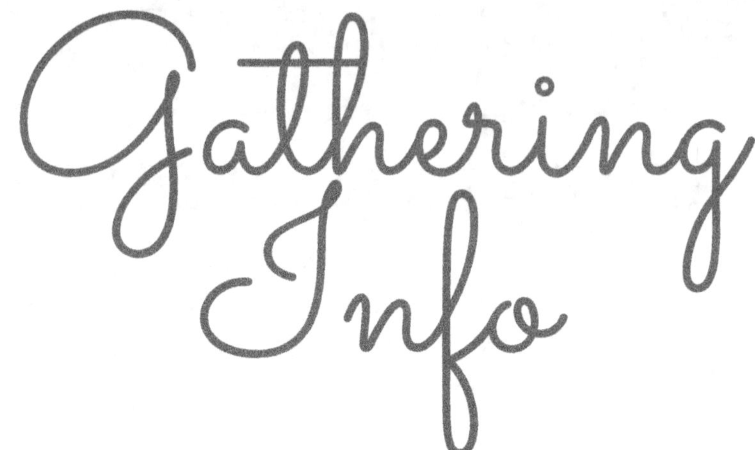

JOT DOWN WORDS ASSOCIATED WITH YOUR HAPPY PLACE
◆ YOU CAN USE SOME OR ALL OF THESE ON THE NEXT PAGE ◆

PLACE:

THINGS YOU SEE

SMELLS

SOUNDS

ALL THE FEELS

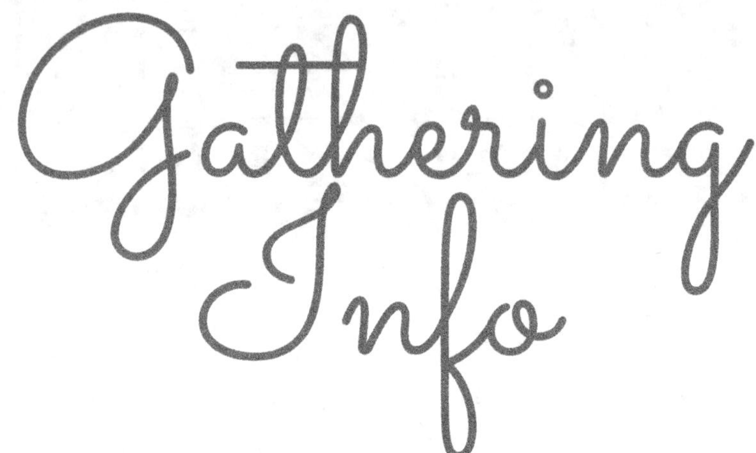

JOT DOWN WORDS ASSOCIATED WITH YOUR HAPPY PLACE
◆ YOU CAN USE SOME OR ALL OF THESE ON THE NEXT PAGE ◆

PLACE:

THINGS YOU SEE

SMELLS

SOUNDS

ALL THE FEELS

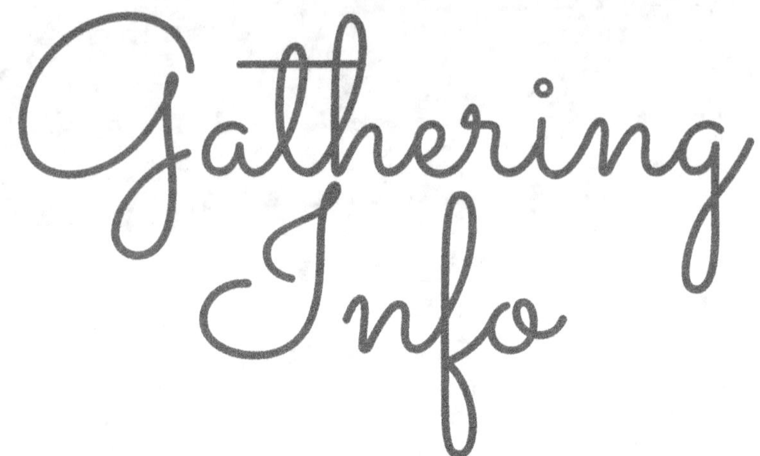

JOT DOWN WORDS ASSOCIATED WITH YOUR HAPPY PLACE
◆ YOU CAN USE SOME OR ALL OF THESE ON THE NEXT PAGE ◆

PLACE:

THINGS YOU SEE

SMELLS

SOUNDS

ALL THE FEELS

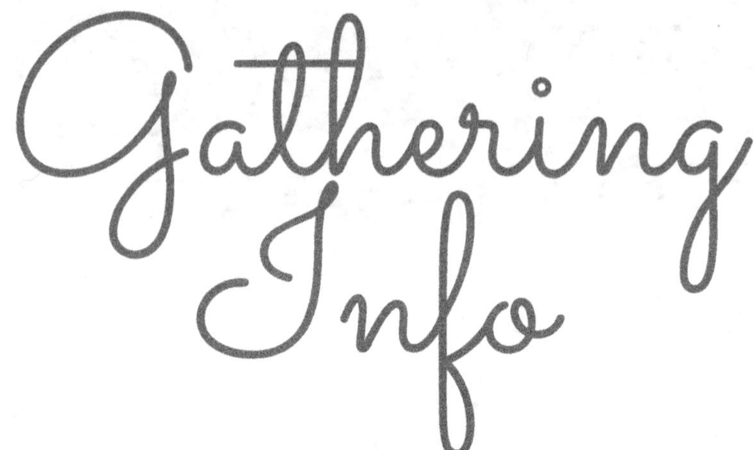

JOT DOWN WORDS ASSOCIATED WITH YOUR HAPPY PLACE
◆ YOU CAN USE SOME OR ALL OF THESE ON THE NEXT PAGE ◆

PLACE:

THINGS YOU SEE

SMELLS

SOUNDS

ALL THE FEELS

One last coloring page

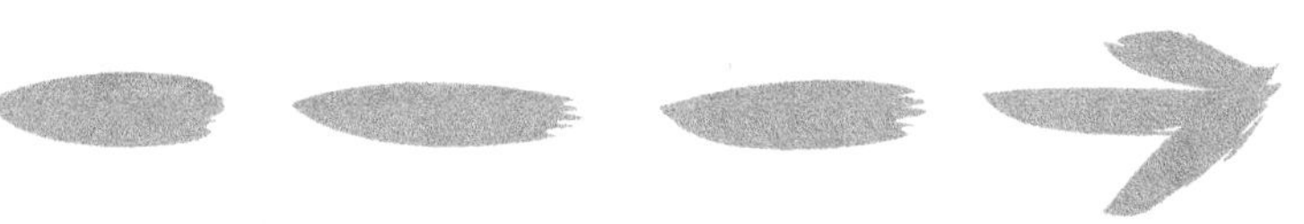

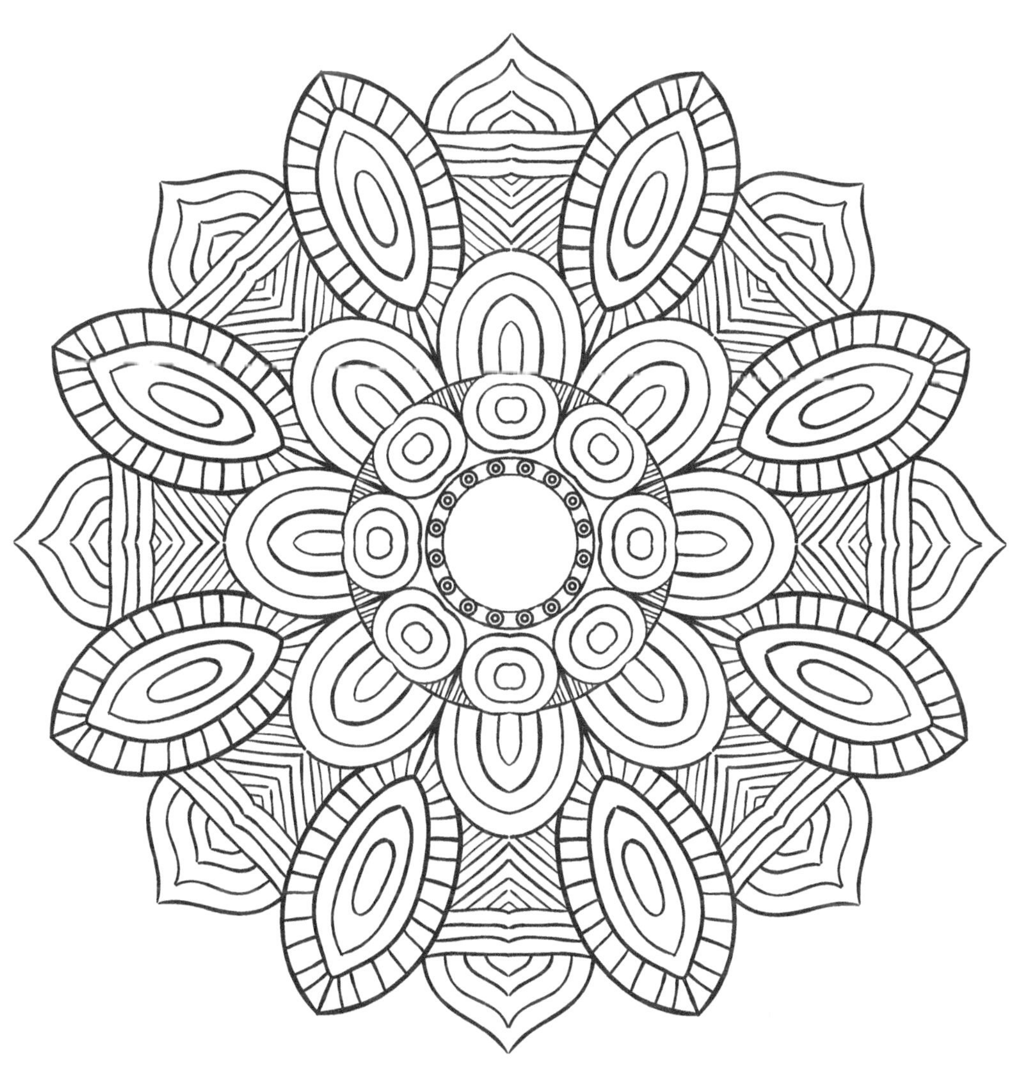

Awesome